Books by Author Bec Filliponi and Illustrator Julie Gebbing

A Very Stressful Day

Peter the Plant and the Big Stormy Cloud
Bailey the Beaver and the Big Stormy Cloud
Maddie the Meerkat and the Big Stormy Cloud
Tess the Turtle and the Big Stormy Cloud

Resource Packs - available for each book
Exploring Therapeutic Concepts with Children

Coming in 2022:
Kevin the Crab Finds His Missing Shell
My Calming Strategies: Regulation Tips for Brilliant Humans
Super Brains and Stressful Days: How EMDR can help us feel less overwhelmed

For more information or to purchase a copy of our books or other resources visit:
Beacon Innovative Solutions - www.beaconis.com.au

This Book Belongs to

____

For my Little People.

You make my world a better place.

A Very Stressful Day

Written by Bec Filliponi.
Illustrated by Julie Gebbing.

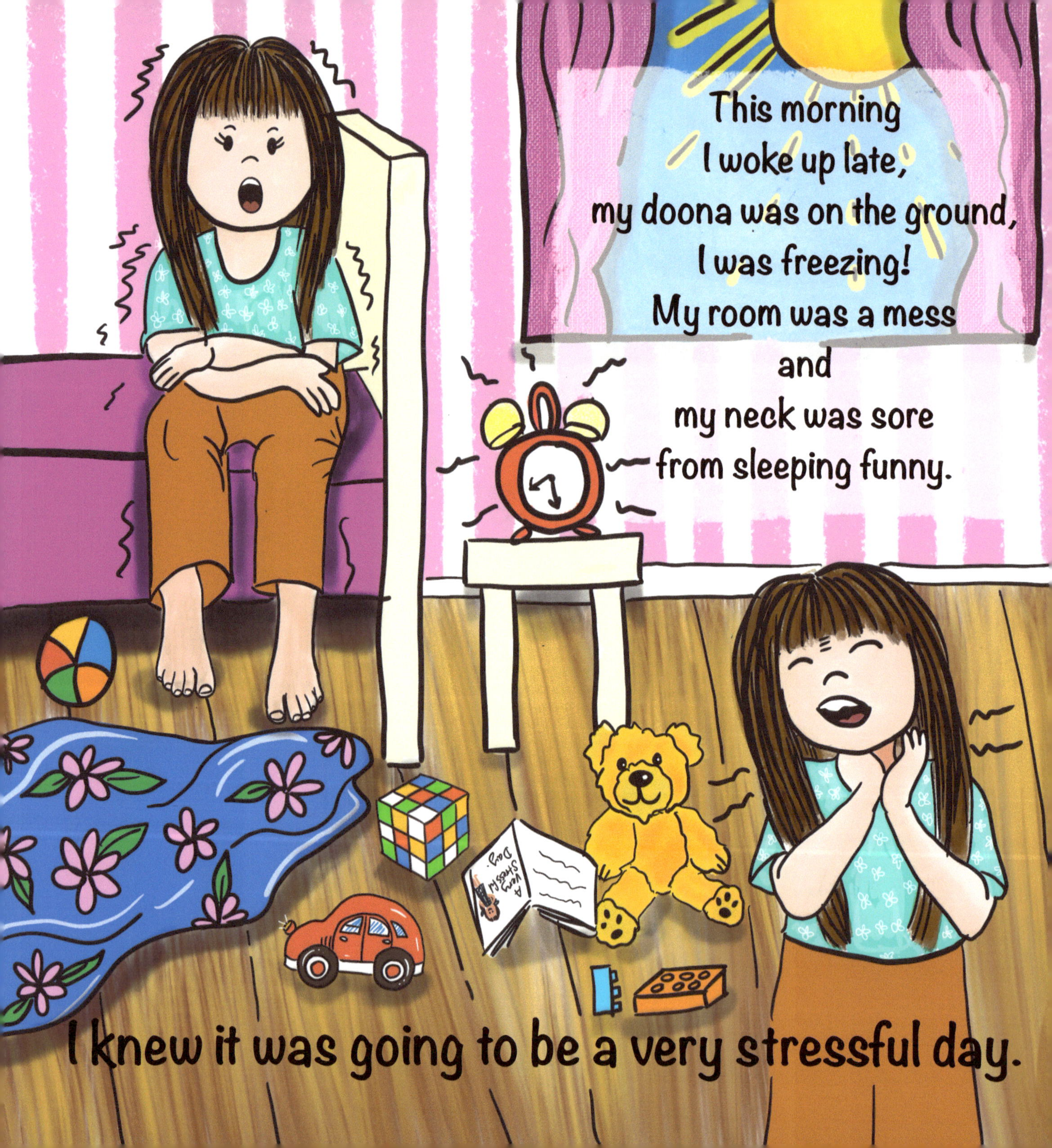

This morning
I woke up late,
my doona was on the ground,
I was freezing!
My room was a mess
and
my neck was sore
from sleeping funny.

I knew it was going to be a very stressful day.

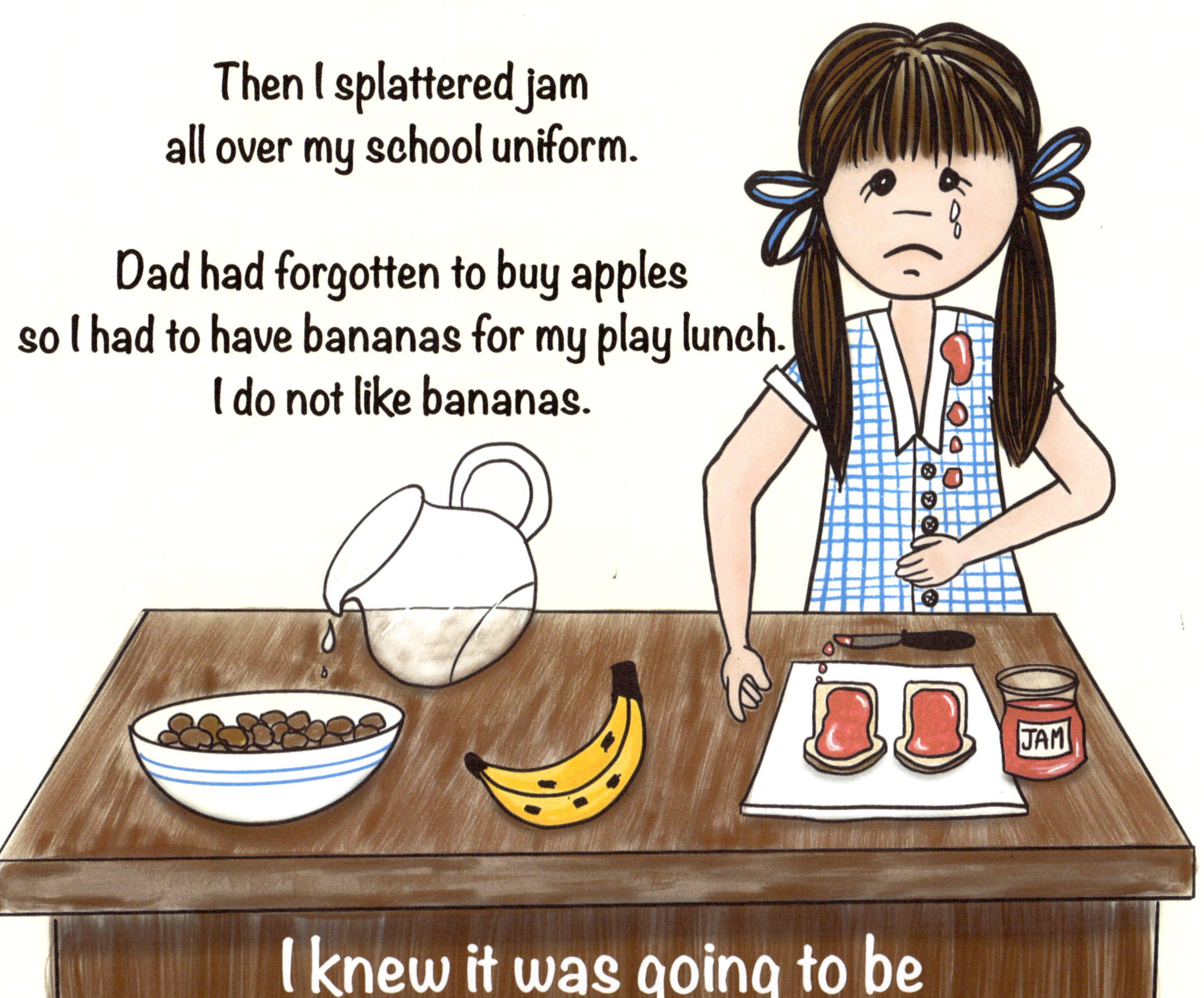

I rushed to the kitchen to eat my breakfast,
but my little sister had used up all the milk.

Then I splattered jam
all over my school uniform.

Dad had forgotten to buy apples
so I had to have bananas for my play lunch.
I do not like bananas.

JAM

I knew it was going to be
a very stressful day.

We had to go to school early because Mum had a work meeting.
It was my turn in the front seat, but my brother raced to the car
and sat there first.
Mum told me to "just sit in the back seat"
which made me very mad because it was my turn
and I felt like no one cared.

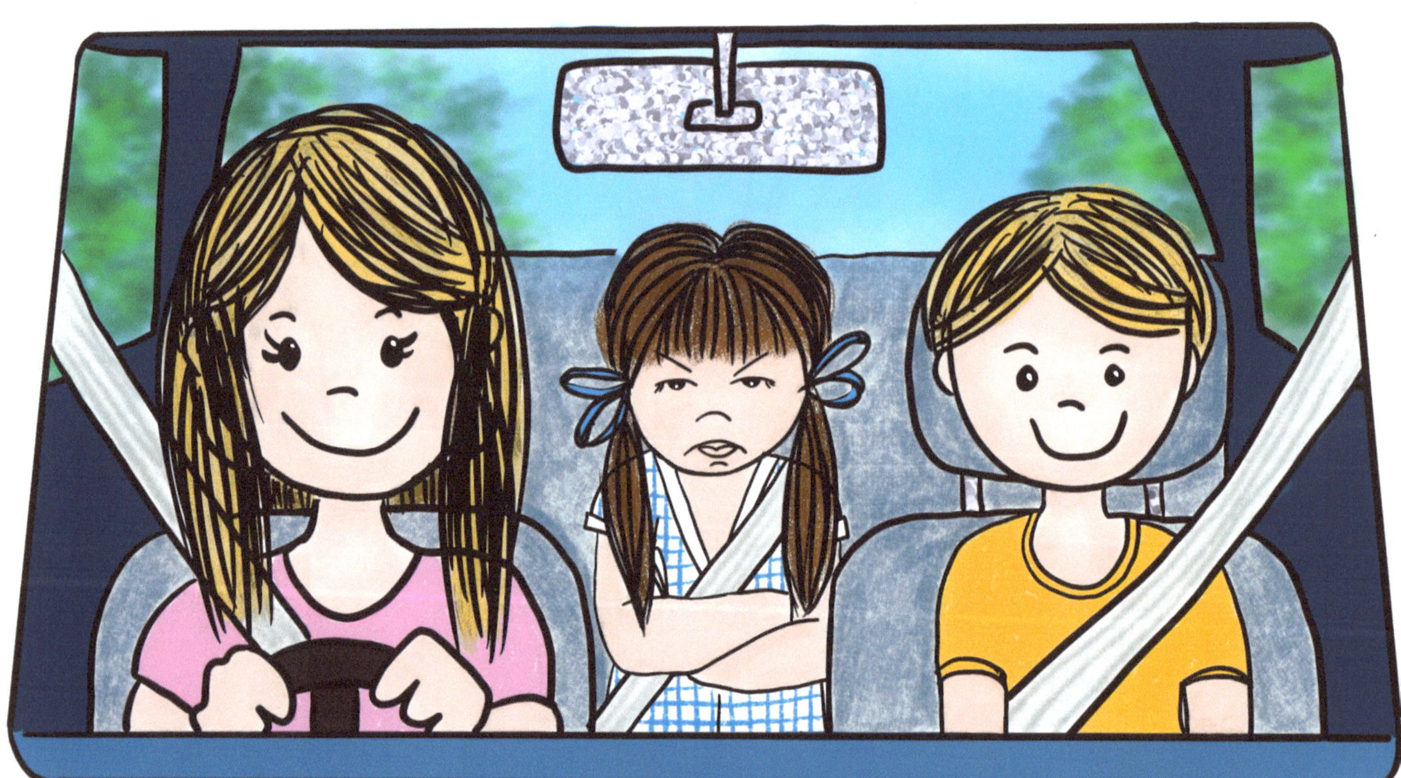

I knew it was going to be a very stressful day.

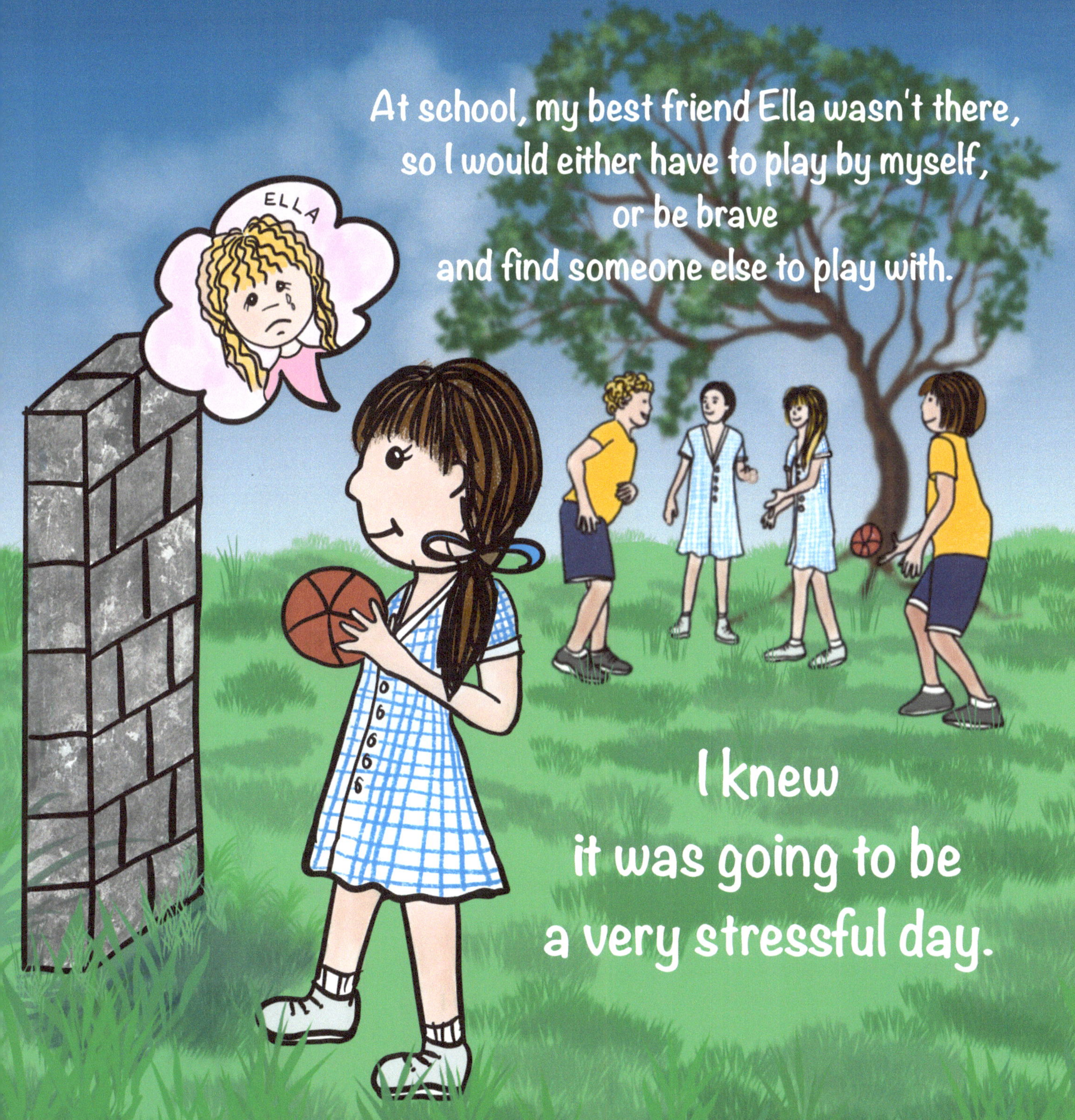

ELLA
At school, my best friend Ella wasn't there,
so I would either have to play by myself,
or be brave
and find someone else to play with.
I knew
it was going to be
a very stressful day.

In my classroom Miss Joey, my teacher,
reminded us that our presentations were today. I hadn't
finished mine, because I didn't understand the last question
and I was really nervous about talking
in front of the whole class.

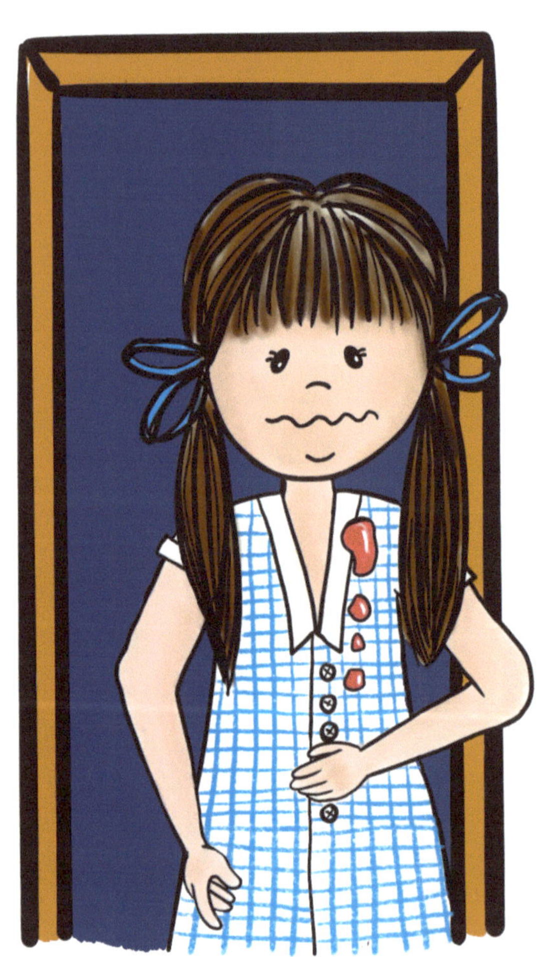

I knew it was
going to be
a very
stressful day.

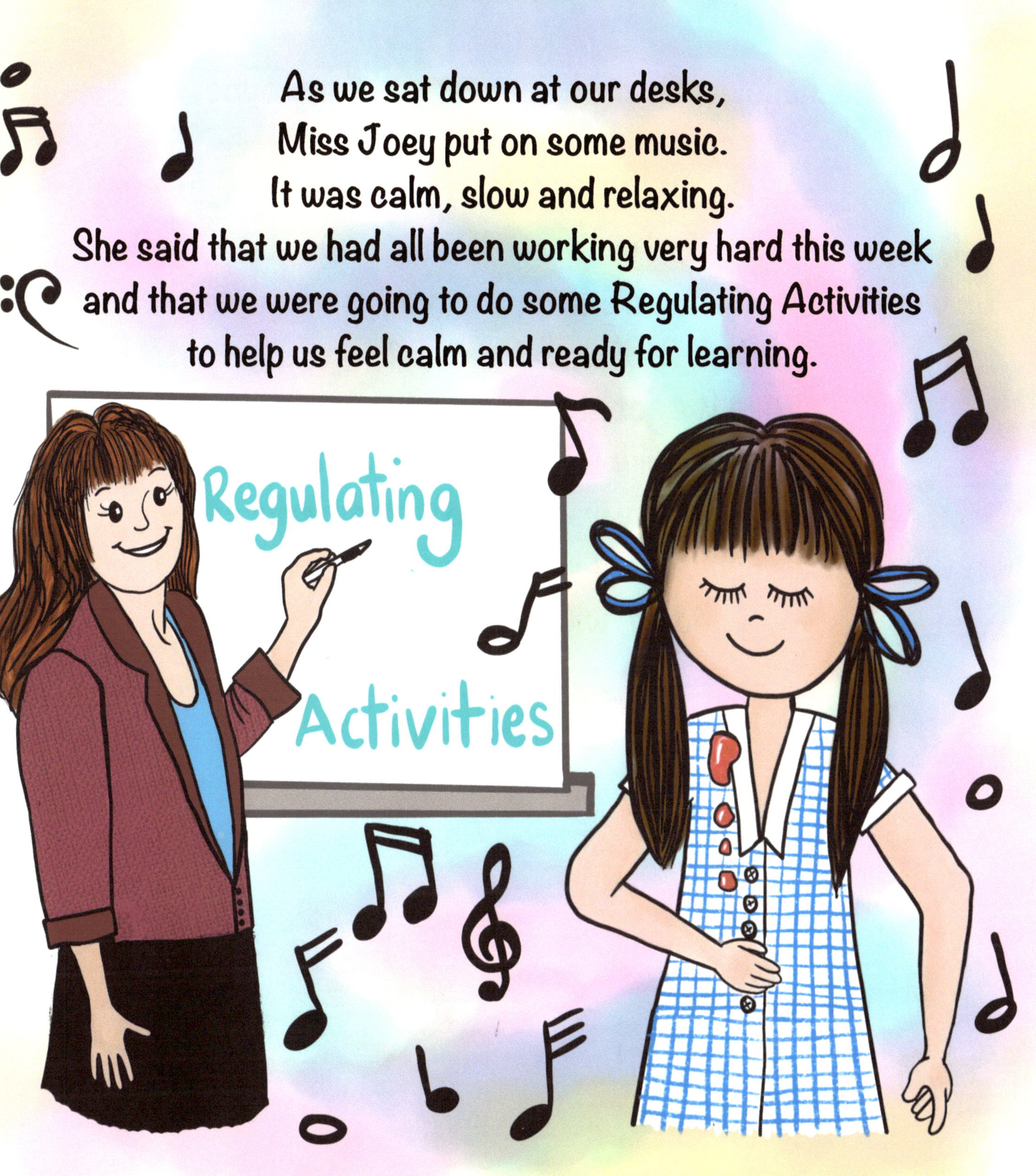

As we sat down at our desks,
Miss Joey put on some music.
It was calm, slow and relaxing.
She said that we had all been working very hard this week
and that we were going to do some Regulating Activities
to help us feel calm and ready for learning.

Regulating

Activities

She told us to push our feet into the ground,
put our hands on our chest
and Breathe in for 1...and out for 1, 2, 3.
She asked us to COUNT COLOURS:
We went around the room saying a number and a different colour.
1 Red, 2 Blue, 3 Green, 4 Pink......
We got all the way up to 14
before we couldn't think of any more colours.
She said if we were doing it by ourselves,
we could count in our heads or out loud,
up to 10, with different colours.

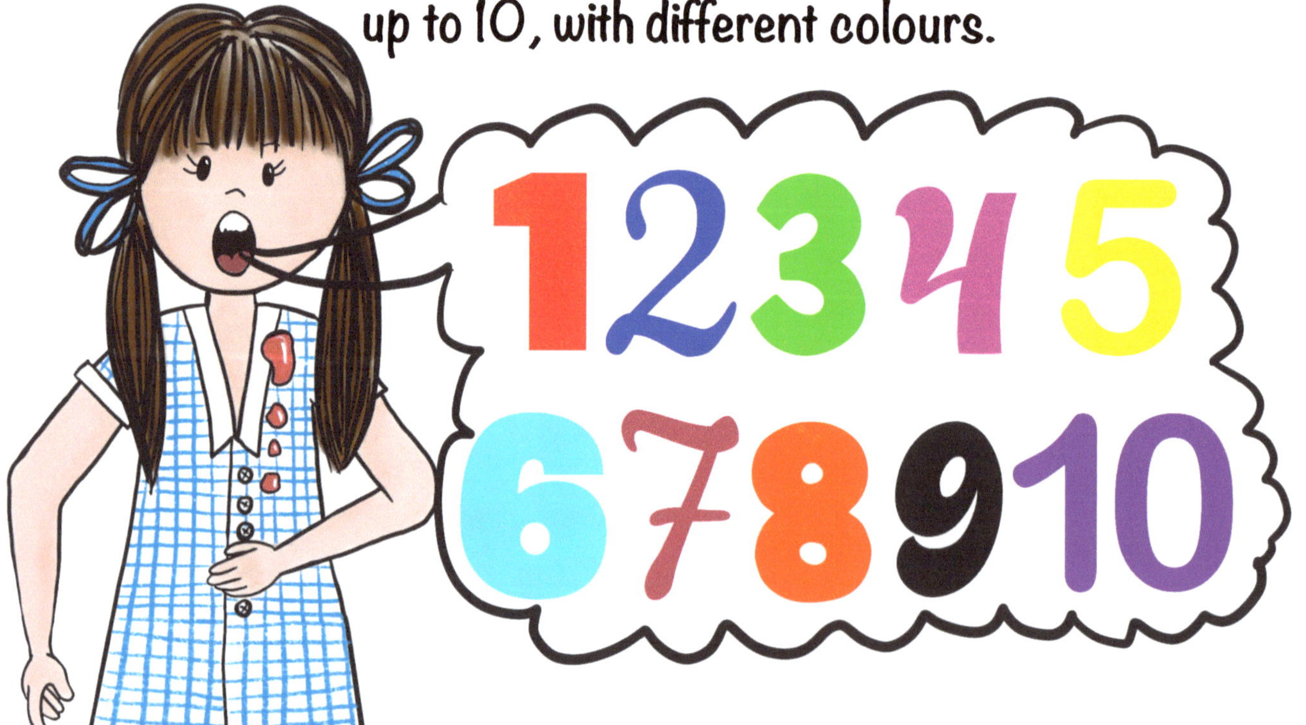

Next she taught us how moving our body either nice and slow,
or fast until we get all puffed out, can help us to Regulate too.
We stood up, rolled our shoulders back 3 times and took a
deep breath in for 1...and out for 1, 2, 3.
Then we stretched up tall to the sky
and let our bodies dangle down like floppy spaghetti.

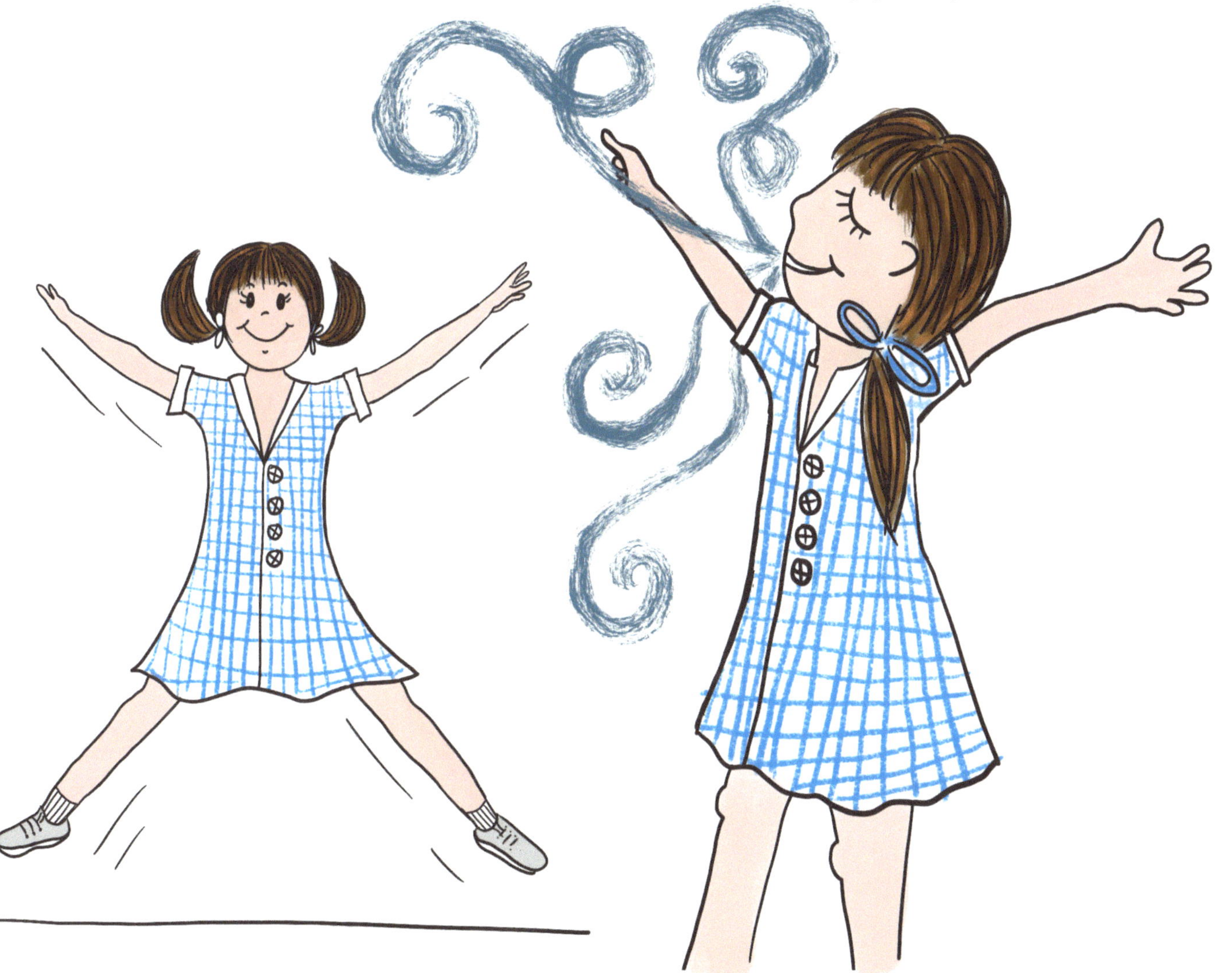

Finally she taught us about Positive Affirmations.
She said that a Positive Affirmation is a statement
that makes our positive belief about ourselves stronger.
It can be anything and if we need some extra ideas,
a friend or family member can help us think of some.

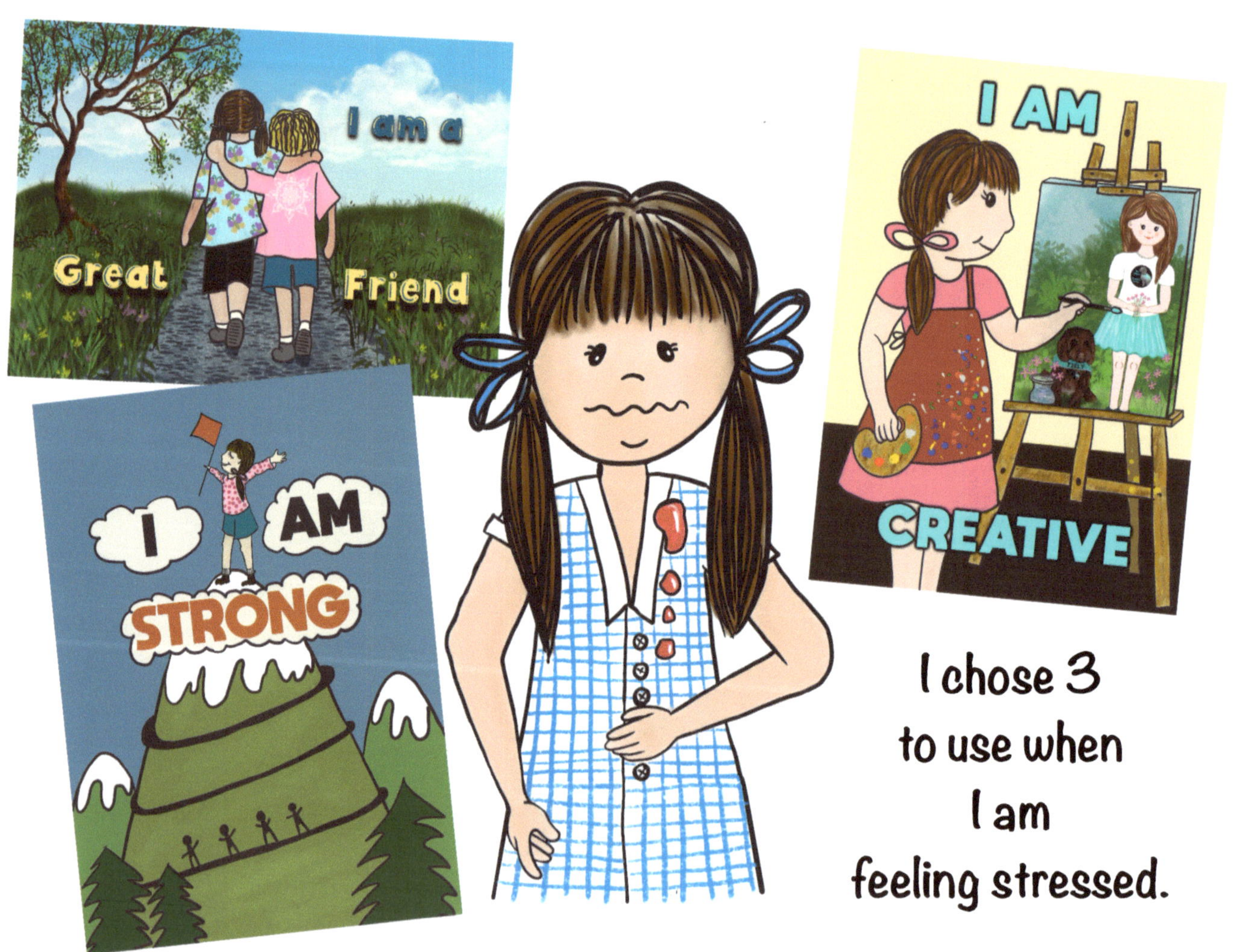

I chose 3
to use when
I am
feeling stressed.

Miss Joey told us
that if we are feeling stressed,
we can talk to her
or another adult we trust
and they can help us
to feel less overwhelmed.

Then we all sat down
and started our next lesson.

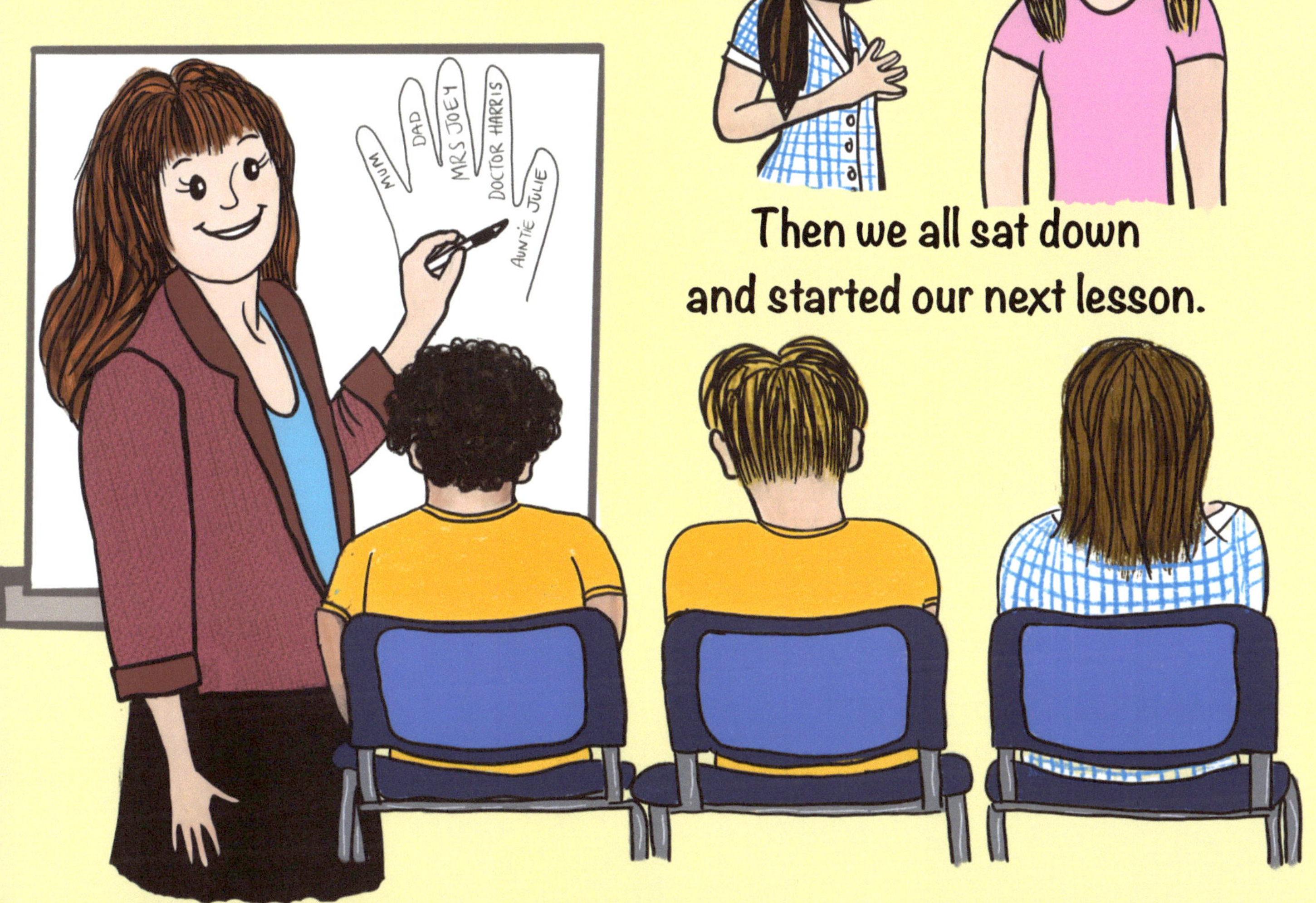

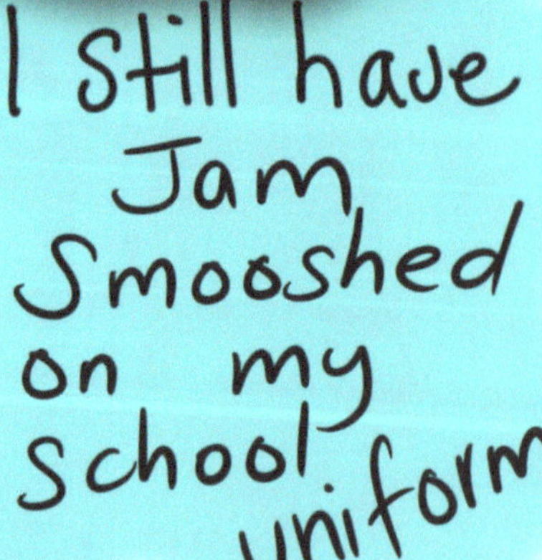

Doing those activities with Miss Joey
and my class got me thinking....

I still have a messy room

I still have Jam Smooshed on my school uniform

I still have a Banana for my lunch

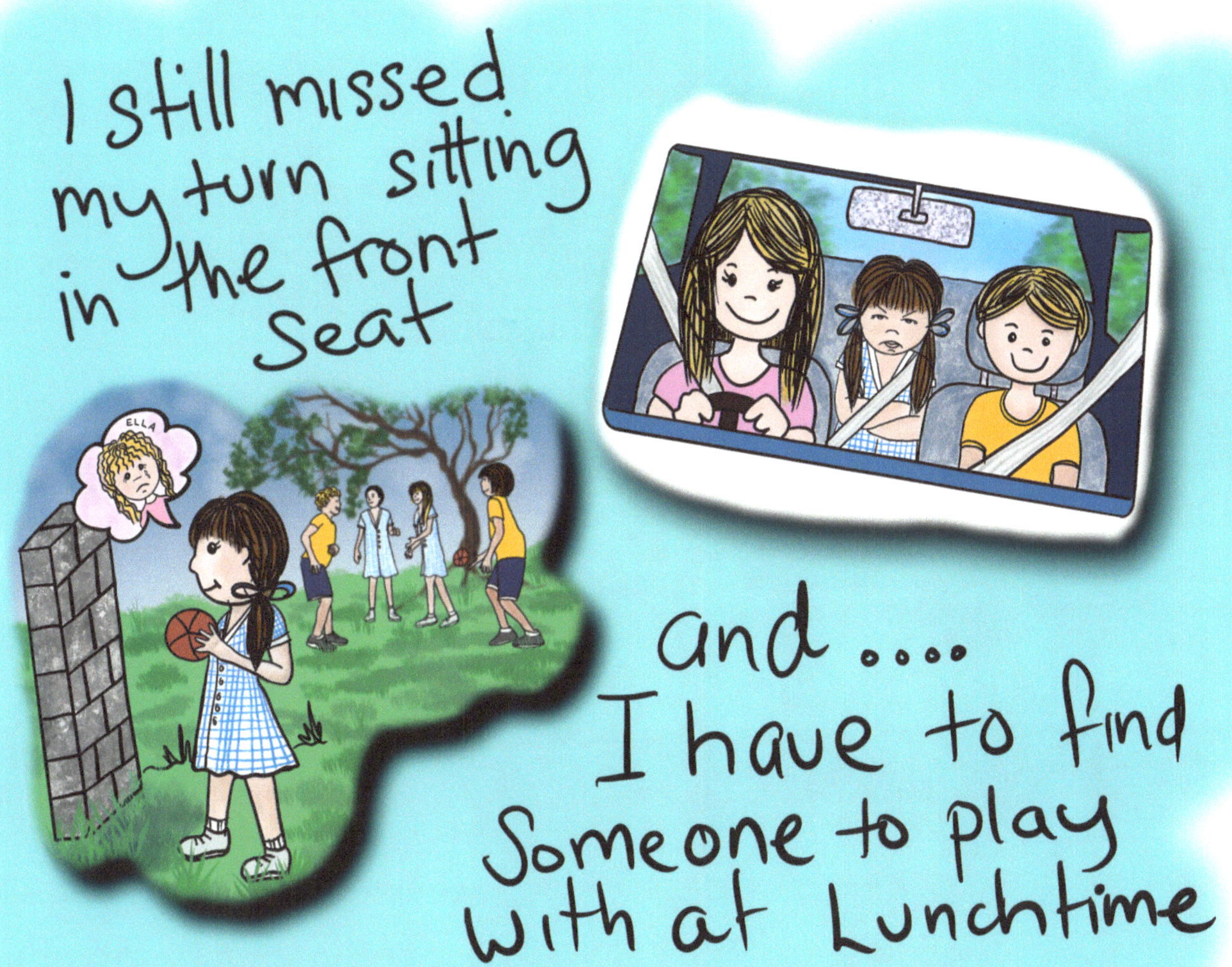

But after doing those Regulating Activities,
I don't feel so overwhelmed
and I don't think
it is going to be such a stressful day after all.

Regulation Strategies

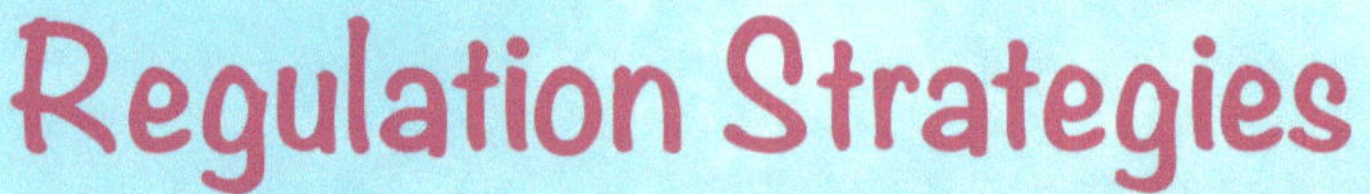

Now that Miss Joey has taught me
how to calm my brain and body,
I can teach you, for your stressful days
and you can teach someone else
for their stressful days.

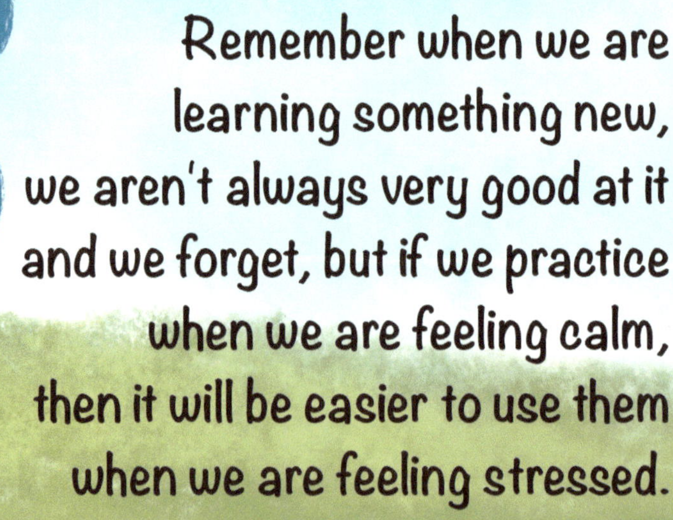

Remember when we are
learning something new,
we aren't always very good at it
and we forget, but if we practice
when we are feeling calm,
then it will be easier to use them
when we are feeling stressed.

Regulation Strategy : Breathing

Our body and our brain are connected.
When our mind and our body are feeling stressed,
breathing helps them to reset
and feel calm and settled again.

Put your feet flat on the ground
and your hands on your chest
like a butterfly.
This helps us feel safe
and connected to our body.
It also helps us to feel our lungs
filling with air
and lets us feel our heart slow down.
Breathe in for 1 and out for 1, 2, 3.
Repeat this 3 times,
or for as long as it takes
for you to feel calmer.

1 Red ♥ 2 Blue ♥ 3 Yellow ♥ 4 Green ♥ 5 Pink ♥ 6 Brown ♥ 7 Turquoise 8 Orange ♥ 9 Magenta ♥ 10 Violet ♥

Regulation Strategy:
Counting Colours

This strategy is good if your stressful thoughts are running really fast,
as it takes your brain power away from your stressful thoughts
and uses it on the Numbers and Colours.
You can do this in your head or out loud.
You can also do this by yourself or
with someone else by taking turns saying the numbers and colours.

Say the numbers 1 to 10
and give each number a different colour:
1 red, 2 blue, 3 orange, 4 purple ....
all the way up to 10.

If you want to make it trickier
you can choose colours all in 1 colour set,
eg: all pinks/reds or all different blues etc.

Regulation Strategy: Roll your shoulders

Slowly roll your shoulders back 3 times, noticing how your body feels as it moves. Now stretch your arms all the way up to the sky, take a breath in and out.

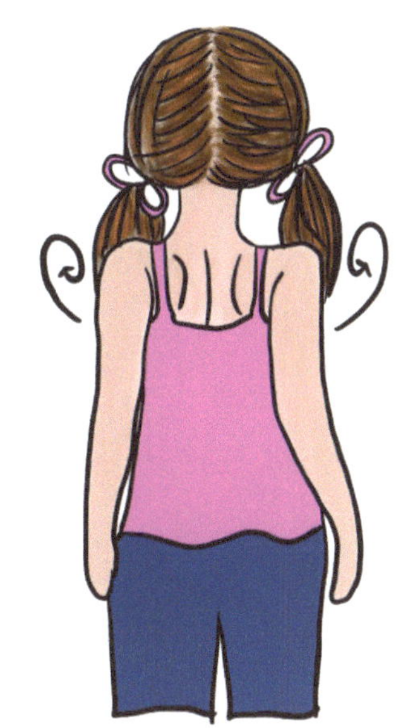

Now bend forward at your waist and let your arms flop to the ground. Notice how your floppy body feels. Is there any tight, loose, sore or relaxed parts? Take a Breath into that part of your body and let it relax, as you breathe out. Slowly unfold back up to standing, rolling your shoulders 3 more times and take a final Breath in for 1 and out for 1, 2, 3.

Regulation Strategy: Positive Affirmations

Positive Affirmations help make our positive feelings about ourselves stronger.
They can be anything.

Start with making a big long list of things that you are good at
or that you like about yourself.
If you find it hard to think of things for yourself,
ask others to help you by telling you all the things
they think are great about you.
Then choose 3 to make into 'I' Statements,
that you think will help you feel positive
and strong when you are stressed or overwhelmed.

Examples:
I am strong, I am creative, I am kind
I am interesting, I try my best, I am smart
I think of ways to do things, I am courageous, I am helpful
I am persistent, I am a good friend, I can do anything
I ask for help when I need it, I am brave, I am thoughtful

Regulation Strategy Tip:

You can pair these strategies together.
You might feel so overwhelmed that you can only just take one breath,
then after a while you might be able to move your body.
You might find it too hard to connect to your body so you might start with Counting
Colours, then move to Breathing, Moving Your Body and finally some Positive
Affirmations to help you feel strong in your new regulated feeling.

Remember we all have stressful days,
but now you have lots of ways
to help you find your calm again.

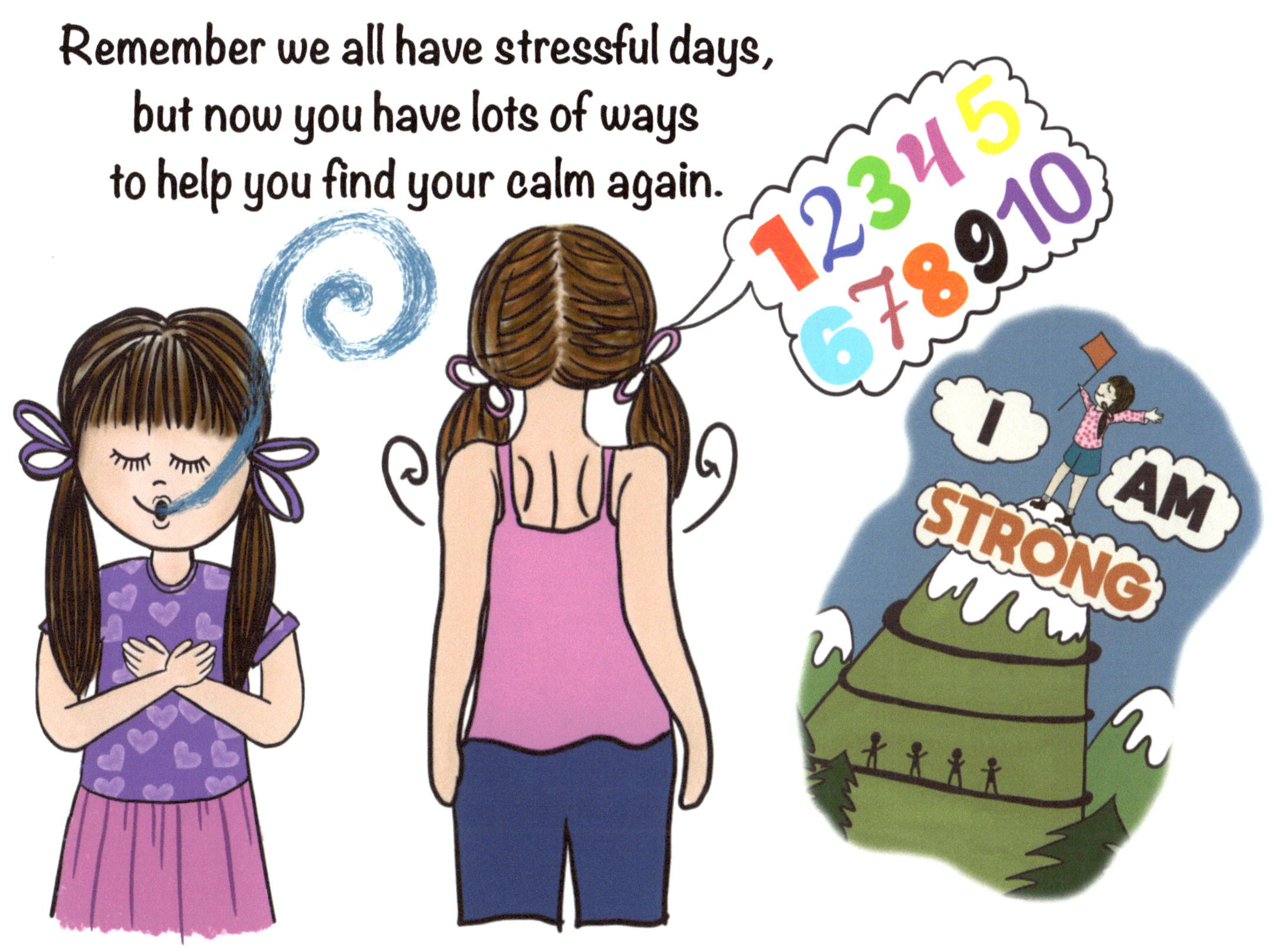

ABOUT THE AUTHOR

Bec Filliponi is an Accredited Mental Health Social Worker, consultant, trainer, author, supervisor and speaker with more then 20 years experience working with children, adolescents, adults and professionals.

Bec specialises in innovative therapies, is EMDR Trained and is an Accredited Animal Assisted Psychotherapist alongside Tilly the Therapy Dog.

She has a degree in Psychology, a degree in Social Work and a Graduate Certificate in Developmental Trauma. Bec has published academic journal articles in the field of social work, is the author of numerous Children's therapeutic story books, therapeutic art journals and has created various therapeutic group programs around violence prevention, early intervention and recovery.

Bec values dignity, accessibility and evidence-based knowledge in her work and specialises in trauma, regulation, mental health, parenting and emotional connection and somatic processing.

ABOUT THE ILLUSTRATOR

Julie Gebbing is an Artist, Photographer and Graphic Designer. She loves all types of Art including Digital Art and is passionate about teaching and inspiring adults and children to be creative. She believes creativity, in all its forms, is an important part of who we are and it can helps us cope with stress and emotions.

Julie studied Art and Graphic Design at Swinburne University and has exhibited her work in many Art & Craft exhibitions. She has run Art and Craft classes for adults and children at her Art Studio and has been involved in the Arts at many local Primary Schools, not-for profit organisations and community projects.

Julie has had a life long dream to illustrate Children's Books and counts it a privilege to fulfill that dream with her daughter Bec. She is proud to create books that help children explore emotions and learn how to regulate and find emotional balance.

**Stressful Days are a normal part of life,
but if you are feeling overwhelmed or feel unsafe,
it is important to talk to an adult or you can call or webchat
a Kids Help Line, where you live.
In Australia contact:**

Kids Help Line   1800 55 1800   kidshelpline.com.au

If your having a stressful day
you can also read the books
from our Big Stormy Cloud Series.

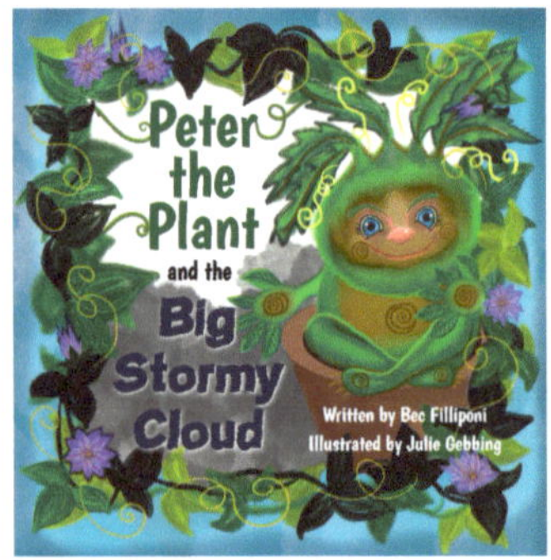

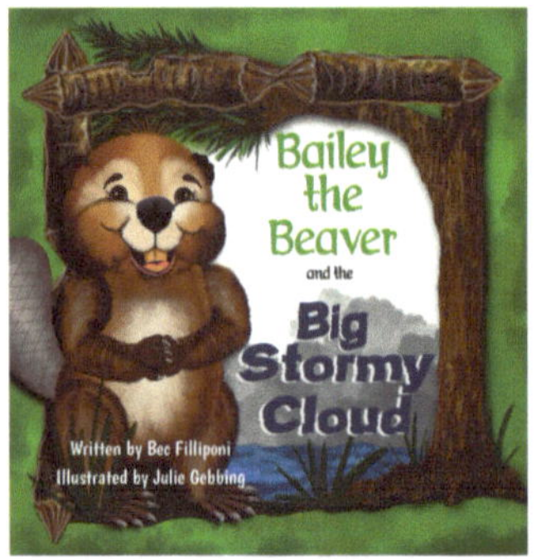

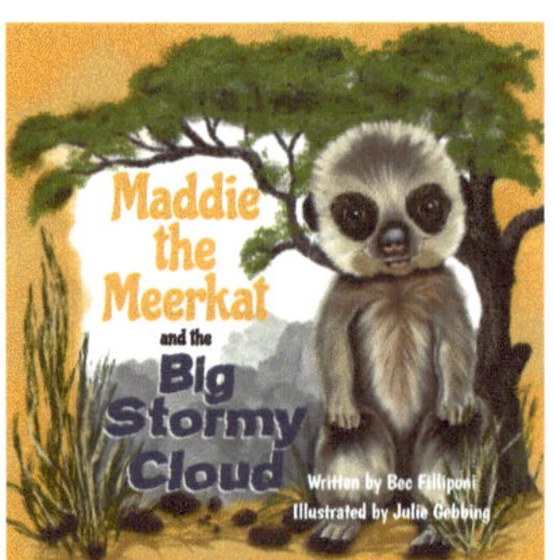

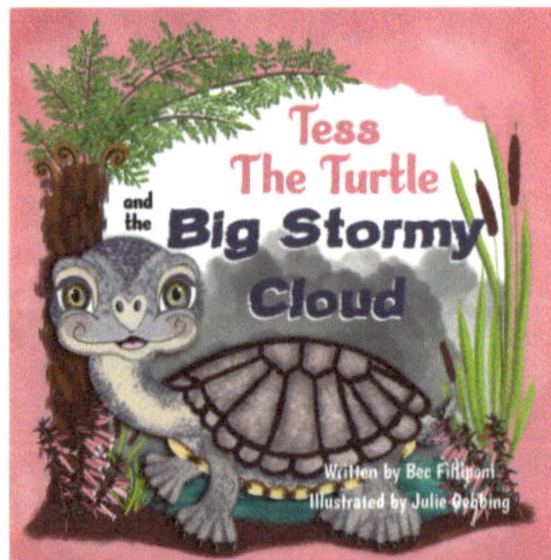

You will find them on our website
www.beaconis.com.au

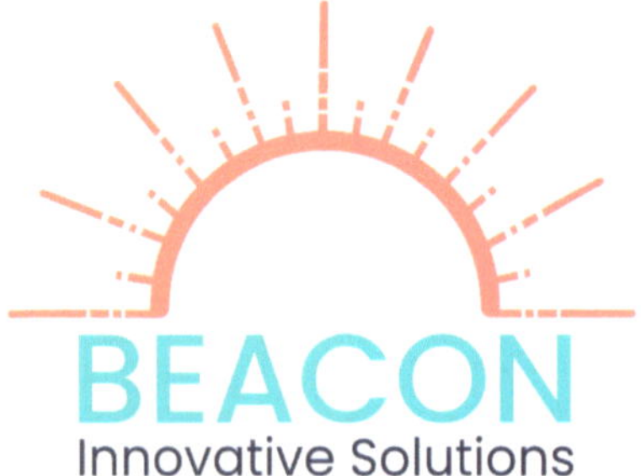